The
Painless Guide
to a
Healthy
Back

The
Painless Guide
to a
Healthy
Back

Ilan
Horowitz
C.A.

Translated by Karen Gold

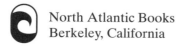
North Atlantic Books
Berkeley, California

The Painless Guide to a Healthy Back

Published by
North Atlantic Books
P.O. Box 12327
Berkeley, California 94701

First English Publication 1991 by Cav-Graph, Jerusalem, Israel

Illustrations by Ellen Horowitz
Photography by P. Horowitz
Cover photograph by Richard Blair
Cover design by Paula Morrison
Printed in the United States of America

The Painless Guide to a Healthy Back is sponsored by The Society for the Study of Native Arts and Sciences, a nonprofit educational corporation whose goals are to develop an educational and crosscultural perspective linking various scientific, social, and artistic fields; to nurture a holistic view of arts, sciences, humanities, and healing; and to publish and distribute literature on the relationship of mind, body, and nature.

Library of Congress Cataloging-in-Publication Data
Horowitz, Ilan.
[Pirke-gav. English]
The painless guide to a healthy back / Ilan Horowitz : translated by Karen Gold.
p. cm. — (Family Healthy Series)
ISBN 1–55643–168–6
1. Backache—Popular works. 2. Backache—Alternative treatment.
3. Medicine, Chinese. I. Title. II. Series.
RD771.B217H6813 1993
617.5'64—dc20   93–11225
                                                      CIP

1 2 3 4 5 6 7 8 9 / 97 96 95 94 93

TABLE OF CONTENTS

to Ellen with love

INTRODUCTION

Back pain can occur for a variety of reasons. These include illnesses that strike at the spinal column and surrounding areas, accidents and emotional stress. Also poor functioning of internal organs such as the kidneys or hereditary defects, excessive stretching of the muscles, and overweight, which place too much strain on the back muscles. Among women, back pain is liable to occur as a result of pregnancy, due to changes and stresses within the skeletal structure. External conditions, such as cold, that block energy and blood flow can also cause painful contractions of the muscles.

In using the term "back pain," I am referring primarily to lower back pain. Treatment for back pain is controversial, in addition to which there are then difficulties in obtaining a precise diagnosis and in identifying the cause. Back pain takes its toll on the sufferer at work, and in the social and emotional spheres of his or her life. Thus a simple everyday task such as dressing, putting on shoes, brushing teeth, sitting down, or even finding a comfortable position for sleeping can turn into a lengthy and painful undertaking. In many cases, back pain leads to feelings of helplessness and depression. As a last resort, many turn to surgery recommended by their doctors, a step that can sometimes even aggravate the existing condition and lead to a state of complete despair.

Most experts in the various medical disciplines agree that the vast majority of back pain occurs as a result of incorrect posture and lack of appropriate physical activity needed to ensure proper maintenance of the spinal column and its supporting muscles. However, even when the cause of the pain is diagnosed as illness or physical trauma, simple exercises — as opposed to more complicated approaches — have proven to be the most effective solution for relieving the pain. The exercises and methods of healing described in this book were developed in the Far East and have been successful over the course of thousands of years in maintaining physical and mental well-being.

Years ago, I suffered a sports-related injury. I was incapacitated and suffered severe back pain. Several different physicians whom I consulted recommended back surgery. I chose not to follow this advice, and instead pursued the approach of traditional Eastern medicine. I now live a pain-free life of physical and mental well-being.

I believe that readers will derive much benefit from this book, and that those who carry out its instructions faithfully are assured of success.

Ilan Horowitz

"Exercise is the key to maintaining good health."

—Maimonides

CHAPTER ONE

THE ANATOMICAL STRUCTURE OF THE SPINAL COLUMN AND CAUSES OF BACK PAIN

The spinal column plays an important role in keeping the body's skeletal structure in an upright position. This function is made possible by the column's unique construction. The three curves of the spinal column give it a somewhat S-shaped appearance. It is this "springy," non-rigid quality that allows the spine to bear the weight of dozens of kilograms.

The spinal column is made up of the following 33 vertebrae: 7 cervical, 12 dorsal, 5 lumbar, 5 sacral, and 4 caudal or coccygeal.

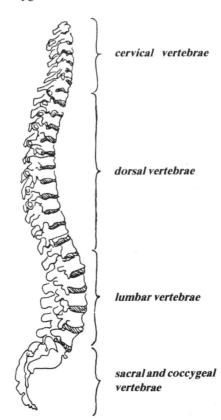

cervical vertebrae

dorsal vertebrae

lumbar vertebrae

sacral and coccygeal vertebrae

Between the vertebrae of the spinal column lie disks composed of elastic cartilage. The purpose of these disks is to separate the vertebrae and allow them to move flexibly. It is the disks that act as "shock absorbers" when our heels come in contact with the ground during walking or running.

In addition to the cartilaginous disks, there are 31 pairs of major nerves located between the spinal vertebrae. These pathways, known as the spinal nerves, are actually clusters that branch out from the spinal cord; which passes through the center of the spinal column and connects to the brain. They emerge from both sides of the spaces that separate the individual spinal vertebrae.

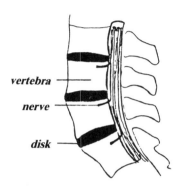

vertebra

nerve

disk

Acute Back Pain

Acute back pain is the result of a hurried or incorrect movement that exerts sudden pressure on a certain portion of the spinal column, causing damage and intense pain, generally in the lower back region. Acute back pain occurs either immediately following the injury to the back or shortly thereafter. Examples of activities likely to cause acute back pain include: working while bent over, falling, lifting heavy objects incorrectly, and performing exercises the wrong way.

Acute back pain is generally experienced as a very sharp pain that prevents us from bending the back either sideways, forward, or backward. Such a condition makes it difficult to walk, to climb stairs, to sit and to lie down; in short, any change of position causes pain. In severe cases of acute back pain, the sufferer needs help in performing even the slightest movement, including simple activities such as dressing and undressing, putting on shoes, or tying shoelaces.

The conventional medical treatment in such cases generally involves bed rest for several weeks accompanied by medication to relieve the pain. Acupuncture and massage treatments, when correctly applied, have proven particularly effective in such cases. They greatly accelerate the healing process and make pain-relief medications unnecessary. One to three acupuncture treatments are usually sufficient to put sufferers back on their feet within 24 to 48 hours of the pain's first occurrence.

Chronic Back Pain

Chronic back pain persists for a lengthy period comprising months or even years. Such pains generally develop from an acute episode of back pain that did not heal properly and, instead, gradually "infiltrated" the body. Chronic back pain can evolve from any of the causes enumerated earlier in this chapter.

The Most Common Forms of Back Pain — Slipped Disk

The spinal column is surrounded by a network of muscles that helps our skeletons remain upright. Intense pressure on the vertebrae brought about by contractions of these muscles, or various other factors such as poor posture, can cause the vertebrae to shift, thus dislocating one or more of the disks located between the vertebrae (a condition often referred to as "slipped disk.") This in turn leads to pressure on one or several of the spinal nerves, resulting in pain.

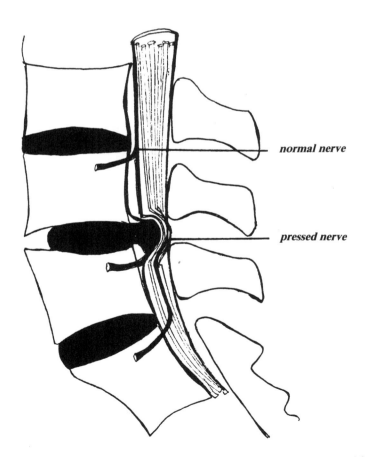

normal nerve

pressed nerve

Sciatica

The sciatic nerve consists of a grouping of spinal nerves emerging from the spaces in between the lumbar and sacral vertebrae, which are located in the lower back region. These nerves come together in the region of the buttocks, from which point the sciatic nerve continues for the full length of the hip and thigh and on down to the ankle. Pressure on one or more of the spinal nerves that comprise the sciatic nerve can cause pain that radiates along the entire length of the nerve. Such pain can reach as far as the knee, or even the ankle.

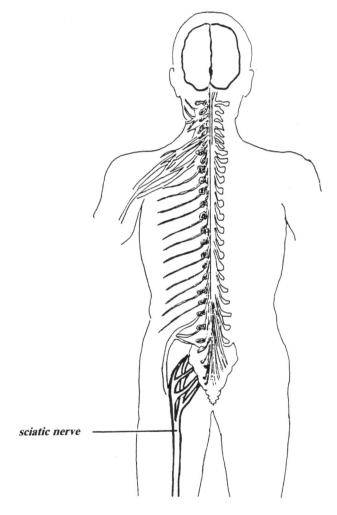

sciatic nerve

A simple method of diagnosing sciatica is to raise the legs straight up toward the ceiling while the patient is lying down. If the patient is suffering from sciatica in a particular leg, he or she will feel pain when that leg is raised even slightly. Sciatica can occur in one or both legs.

CHAPTER TWO

BACK PAIN IN CHINESE MEDICINE
Meridians, Energy, and Acupuncture Points

Our bodies house energy channels (meridians) through which our life energy flows. This energy is known in Chinese as qi (pronounced "chee"). Every internal organ in the body possesses its own energy channel, with the primary energy channels totalling fourteen in number.

Each energy channel has both an external and an internal path. The external path passes along the surface of the skin and through the muscles of the body, and contains the points used during acupuncture, while the internal path of each channel connects it to the internal organ with which it is associated and to additional channels and organs. Together, these form an invisible network of channels which can be compared to an array of spider webs.

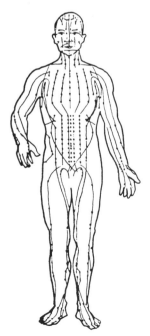

The Meridians on the front of the body

The Internal and the External in Chinese Medicine

In Chinese medicine, the internal and the external are linked with one another; what lies inside finds expression on the outside (as pain, sensitivity, various feelings, etc.). Treatment conducted on the outside produces effects on the inside as well, for they are one. The body and soul are intertwined: Acupuncture at the points situated over the area requiring treatment, or at points in other locations on the body, affects the problem area through the complicated network of energy channels. Chinese medical treatment is primarily external in nature; however, it focuses on central points that affect the inside of the body.

Pain is viewed as stemming from a blocked, or otherwise impaired, flow of energy through the meridians. Pain relief treatment therefore involves the "opening" of these energy channels so as to allow the resumption of unimpeded flow. This constitutes the guiding principle of practitioners of this method.

According to Chinese medicine, a health problem indicates a state of disharmony in the body's energy. This state, whose origins may lie in various factors — some external and some internal — is characterized either as one of "excess" or of "deficiency" (weakness). An "external" state is generally one of excess, and usually expresses itself as acute pain stemming from an accident or a dislocation of the vertebrae. (Such a state may sometimes be brought on by external factors as well, such as the weather, specifically humidity or cold that penetrates the body.) An "internal" state, on the other hand, is generally one of weakness or deficiency.

Because the kidneys are situated in the lower back region, a deficiency in the energy activity of this organ often plays a strong role in lower back pain. Particularly in the case of chronic back pain of long duration, it is safe to assume the presence of a state of weakness of some type in the kidneys. Chinese medicine's flexible approach holds that an external state can become an internal one, and vice versa. The practitioner of Chinese medicine will generally refer to an internal problem involving lower back pain as a deficiency of the kidneys' yang or yin.

Classic Division of Types of Back Pain According to Chinese Medicine

Without entering into a complex explanation of the energy qualities known as yin and yang, the following table offers a partial breakdown of the most common types of back pain as viewed by traditional Chinese medicine:

Cause	Chinese Definition	Symptoms
External	Back pain as result of external injury	Sharp back pain resulting from a fall, incorrect movement, or lifting heavy objects. Pain greatly impedes movement. State can be acute or chronic.
Internal	Deficiency — kidneys' yang	Deep, dull pain and sensation of cold in lower back; weakness in knees; rapid onset of fatigue upon exertion; pale, shiny face; frequent nocturnal urination; salty taste in mouth; dark bags under the eyes; diminished sexual energy.
Internal	Deficiency — kidney's yin	Deep, dull pain in lower back; weakness in knees; ringing in ears; dizziness; insomnia. Condition worsens in afternoon and evening.
External & internal	Humidity	Lower back pain, worsening under humid conditions; feeling of heaviness in head & limbs; frequent expellation of urine in small amounts.

Traditional Chinese Methods of Treatment for Back Pain

Acupuncture: This treatment entails neural stimulation at prescribed acupuncture points. Such stimulation can be performed by assorted techniques involving needles, suction cups, or the application of heat (generated by burning an herb known as moxa) to the various points.

Exercises: The practitioner guides the patient through a series of pain relief exercises. Many of the exercises that appear in this book are also practiced by the Chinese for relief of back pain.

Manipulations: This method is actually very similar to that of a chiropractor who "restores" the bones to their proper position. Such manipulations ease the pressure exerted on the spinal nerves.

Medicinal Herbs: Practitioners treating a weakness in the kidneys, for example, have at their disposal specific herbs for strengthening the kidneys, in accordance with the patient's particular type of weakness. Cinnamon is one of the primary medicinal herbs in Chinese medicine. Back pain is numbered among the many conditions that it can alter. Cinnamon also possesses the attribute of "warming and strengthening" the kidneys. When used for this purpose, it is employed in greater amounts than in its role as a spice.

Massage (Shiatsu): This is a method of pressing the fingers on the acupuncture points. Such pressure can relax the muscles in the painful area, release tensions, and restore energy flow (qi) in the region of the pain.

The above-mentioned forms of treatment can be integrated, and are not mutually exclusive.

Direct Effect of the Acupuncture Points on the Internal Organs

The spinal nerves are connected to the internal organs. Pressure on one or more of these nerves can inhibit the passage of neural messages to the related organs, potentially causing pain as well as impairing the functioning of these organs. Pain does not always occur in such cases: there may be impaired functioning with no pain present, or a state of pain with no other problems.

The spinal nerves at the lower portion of the spinal column are related to the urinary tract and the reproductive organs. The lower back is situated in the middle of the body — site of an important energy center. For this reason, it is inevitable that urinary tract problems, impaired sexual functioning, and strong overall fatigue will appear in concert with lower back pain.

Major acupuncture points are situated directly over the associated spinal nerves on both sides of the spinal column, along its full length. By treating these points, the pressure on these nerves is reduced, thus permitting the qi (energy) to flow properly. This achieves the dual purpose of relieving pain and improving the functioning of the internal organs.

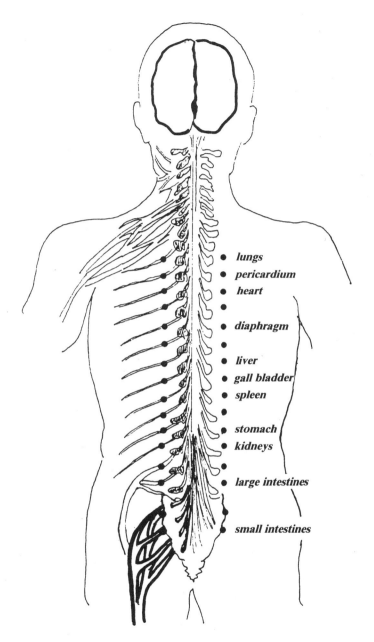

Relationship of acupuncture points to the spinal nerves and internal organs

CHAPTER THREE

PHYSICAL ACTIVITY: EAST AND WEST

Insufficient physical activity is one of the causes of energy disharmony and physical, as well as mental, illness. This connection was already known to the ancients of both the East and West. The Greeks, in the West, concluded from this the need to develop the body's muscles, while the Orient adopted a different approach which stressed flexibility of the body. These contrasting approaches still characterize the two cultures today.

Physical Activity in the West: Strength and Speed

In the Western nations, physical activity is based on competition and on strenuous use of the muscles through rapid, dynamic movements. This approach is very effective in our early years. A young person, full of energy and vitality, and still growing and developing, is capable of almost unlimited, arduous physical activity.

Sports such as running, weightlifting, wrestling, and gymnastics of various types do provide an outlet for emotional tension and improve the body's health, but this approach also contains a number of drawbacks:

a. When performing strenuous activities, the body loses energy, making rest periods a necessity.

b. There is a risk of damage to the vertebrae, tendons, and muscles caused by such activities.

c. These activities are limited to young people.

d. Performing such activities can cause pain.

e. The competitive factor "poisons" the attitude of participants in such sports, and can sometimes increase tension instead of relieving it.

Physical Activity in the East:
Flexibility and Energy Flow

The Eastern approach to physical activity differs completely from that of the West. In the first place, Eastern attitudes in this area are opposed to the competitive component. Here, the competition is an internal one; it is waged only between the person performing the activity and him or herself.

The energy channels (meridians) involved in Chinese medicine pass under the skin and through the muscles. They are connected to the tendons, the blood vessels, and the nervous system. We can compare an energy channel to a rubber hose: when the hose is flexible and strong, water flows through it smoothly; but when the hose is bent, after being stored unused for too long a time, it becomes rigid, loses its flexibility, and functions poorly.

The same holds true for muscles and tendons that have become inflexible as a result of insufficient activity (or, alternatively, because of over-development, as in the case of the body builder).

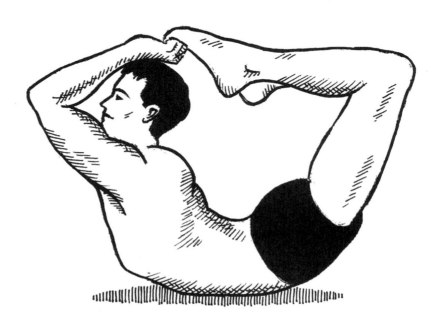

The meridians and blood vessels undergo the same phenomenon as the neglected rubber hose. Energy flow is impeded, producing a negative effect on that person's health. In light of the above, it becomes clear that for our bodies' long-term best interests, flexibility exercises performed according to Eastern methods are preferable to strengthening exercises and "inflated" muscle development.

The following is a list of the advantages of Eastern forms of exercise which originated in India and China (such as yoga and tai qi*):

a. The emphasis in performing these exercises is on acquiring flexibility.
b. The exercises do not cause loss of energy; rather, they increase the body's energy level. Instead of feelings of fatigue, they generate a sense of alertness and calm.
c. They carry no danger of physical harm.
d. They have a "softening" emotional effect, and can even help ease emotional problems.
e. They retain body flexibility and proper energy flow through the various meridians.
f. They have a definite positive effect on the internal organs, such as the heart, kidneys, lungs, liver, and others.
g. They do not cause pain.
h. They provide us with a measure of assurance of long life.
i. Since the element of competition is absent, there is no emotional wear and tear.
j. These exercises can also be performed at an advanced stage in life.

---

* Tai qi is a system of exercises, developed in China, whose aim is to circulate the energy (qi) in the meridians. Yoga exercises, which originated in India, have a similar goal.

CHAPTER FOUR

AGE, FLEXIBILITY AND GOOD HEALTH
The body's vitality depends on flexibility —
not on muscle strength

Infants and children possess flexible bodies, a factor which prevents them from suffering chronic pain. The reason for this, according to Chinese medicine, is that in a flexible body the qi (energy) flows unimpeded, thus allowing the body to function efficiently and without pain.

As people age, the flexibility of their body decreases, resulting in a disruption of the qi's proper flow through the energy channels (meridians) that pass through the muscles. For example, most people find it difficult, as early as age 40, to touch their toes without bending their knees. A disturbance in the flow of the qi increases the likelihood that pain and other health problems will occur.

The majority of people between the ages of 30 and 35 do not suffer from special health problems, even if they do not engage in regular physical activity. That is because, up until this point, the body is naturally strong. Beyond this age, regular physical activity becomes extremely important for the proper maintenance of the body.

It is widely known that people who exercise regularly and retain their flexibility enjoy energy, vitality and good health even into their senior years.

Women possess a higher degree of flexibility than men, and also enjoy a longer life expectancy, facts which would indicate a possible connection between flexibility and the length of our lives.

Flexibility of the body, then, maintains the proper flow of the qi through the energy channels, thus preventing pain and other health problems. It should be noted that the unimpeded flow of the qi through the body also aids in the functioning of the internal organs.

Many people have the mistaken impression that their bodies do not need exercise because their daily work routine involves at least some exertion and, at times, even great physical effort. However, in most types of labor, the worker does not perform the full range of movements for which the body is designed. The result of neglecting to perform exercises aimed at promoting flexibility on a regular and consistent basis is the gradual degeneration of the tendons, muscles and joints. This in turn leads to difficulties when the

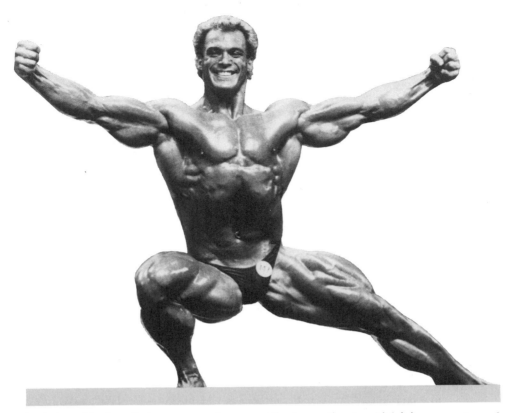

body is suddenly called upon to perform a particular motion to which it is unaccustomed. The same holds true for those who regularly engage in sports whose major purpose is to develop and "inflate" the muscles of the body. Such 'body builders' are limited in their ability to perform even relatively simple stretching exercises.

The body of the athlete pictured here is attractive and well-developed, but his joints and muscles are incapable — due to their exaggerated dimensions — of performing the entire gamut of movements for which they were intended. In contrast, a slender person whose muscles are more relaxed, and less tense and "inflated," will be able to perform a wider variety of stretching exercises with greater ease.

Warm-up exercises, which for the most part are actually various forms of stretching, are essential before engaging in sports. These exercises are commonly performed **before** the activity in order to enhance one's physical abilities. When stretching exercises are attempted following vigorous exertion of the muscles and **after** the body has "cooled down," there is a certain degree of difficulty because the strenuous activity has caused the muscles to contract and to lose their flexibility.

Performing a stretching exercise of even the simplest kind causes the body to incorporate the new movement. Doing this same exercise on a regular basis helps the body become accustomed to the movement and to perform it with increased ability.

When a particular movement is not performed repeatedly and consistently, this process of adjustment is transformed into one of decline. **From this we learn the vital importance of regular daily exercise aimed at enhancing the body's flexibility.**

CHAPTER FIVE

SEXUAL ACTIVITY AND BACK PAIN
Sexual Activity as a Factor in the Recovery Process

"The yellow emperor asked: 'I have heard that the ancients often lived to be one hundred and remained as if still in their youth, while in our day, when we reach the age of fifty, our activity diminishes. Why is this? For what reason?'
And the wise doctor Chi Pu answered:
'The ancients knew the way (tao) and the laws of the yin and yang. They understood the importance of living in harmony with nature... but today we do not act in this way... and because of our sexual desires and our incessant sins against nature, we have lost the 'truth.'"

From: "Classic Internal Medicine of the Yellow Emperor", 2674 B.C.E.

Sexual activity is touted time and again as a method of relieving or preventing back pain. This claim is based on the fact that the sex act involves use of the back muscles, thereby presumably strengthening them. Scientific research also shows that sexual activity stimulates the release of endorphine hormones, which are similar in their chemical composition to the pain-relieving drug morphine. But the supposed beneficial effects of sexual activity on back pain are negated by modern reality. We see an extremely high incidence of back pain specifically among the 20-plus age group, which engages in regular sexual activity.

Chinese medicine, which preaches a lifestyle that is in harmony with nature, stresses that excessive sexual activity weakens the body and is liable to hinder its recovery process. The importance of the activity of the kidneys should be understood within this context.

The *jing*, or life energy, is concentrated primarily in the kidneys. It constitutes the major energy force in the life processes of our bodies from the moment of birth, extending through all the stages of growth and development. This is the energy that helps the body to overcome injury and recover from illness. And it is this same force that creates life and ensures its perpetuation through the processes of conception and birth.

The *jing* is, in reality, our sexual energy. Every person is allocated a specific amount of this energy: over the course of our lives, we draw our *jing* from these reserves. If this were not the case, we would remain young till the end of our days. In men, the *jing*'s depletion is accelerated by the act of ejaculation, while in women, pregnancy produces the same effect.

The power of our sexual energy is awesome. Consequently, during our process of recovery from illness or injury, we should marshall this force for the purpose of overcoming pain and weakness. This truth is accepted by Chinese medicine, just as it was by the ancient physicians of the West, the bearers of the Hippocratic oath. Maimonides, a religious scholar and physician, taught the laws of life through his writings. In his work entitled *Mishneh Torah* (*Sefer Hamada*, Chapter IV), he describes the importance of the body's sexual energy : **"The semen is the life force of the body... the more it is expended, the more the body is weakened and its strength diminished... and many pains... occur."** It is necessary, therefore, for men suffering from back pain to moderate their sexual activity, **especially if the discomfort is accompanied by symptoms of weakness in the kidneys.** For women, sexual activity does not constitute an impediment to the process of recovery.

CHAPTER SIX

NATURAL TREATMENTS FOR RELIEF OF BACK PAIN

In addition to exercises, there are other methods of treatment for relief of chronic or acute back pain that can speed up the recovery process. Practiced for centuries, these natural forms of treatment have demonstrated their effectiveness in relieving pain and improving overall health.

During an acute attack, the intensity of the back pain can sometimes be so great that the person suffering is incapable of performing even the smallest movement. In such a case, the only option is to have another person administer treatment. The methods which we shall examine here are: massage (shiatsu), suction cups, compresses, and reflexology. These forms of treatment are capable of relieving back pain, and carry the added benefit of enhancing the patient's overall state of health.

Such "alternative" medical treatments bear a distinct advantage over the methods of conventional medicine: while the former are relatively harmless and will not aggravate the existing condition, the latter may inflict damage and even bring about further deterioration. In light of the above, it is my belief that alternative methods should be preferred over conventional approaches when selecting methods of treatment for back pain. Moreover, alternative approaches can be practiced independently at home, with the aid of a friend or relative.

The following is a description of the techniques used in natural treatments for the relief of back pain. These methods are simple and effective, and anyone can apply them by following the instructions provided below. The effectiveness of the treatments increases with greater practical experience.

The patient must undergo a full medical examination before beginning these treatments in order to ascertain if there is an underlying condition that might render such methods inappropriate. Pregnant women should not be treated by laymen since pregnancy is a unique natural state of disharmony: unskilled attempts to channel the body's energy flow by means of acupuncture, shiatsu or reflexology run the risk of inducing premature labor and spontaneous abortion.

Massage (Shiatsu)

Massage and pressure (shiatsu) on the classic acupuncture points scattered over the body bring about relief from pain. The massage is performed by pressing a finger (generally the thumb) in a circular motion over the points selected. A medium degree of pressure should be applied — not hard enough to produce pain but not too light either. The duration of the pressure varies according to the number of points chosen and the length of the treatment session.

During the treatment, cooperation between the practitioner and the patient is a necessity. The latter must guide the former as to when and where to step up or to lessen the pressure being applied to the various points. In addition, there will be regions where the patient experiences particularly intense relief during the course of treatment. It is advisable to linger over these spots for a longer period.

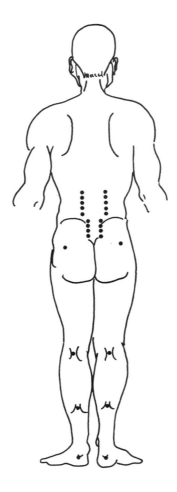

Pressure points for relief of back pain

Friction Massage (Heat Massage)

In this massage technique, oil (preferably olive or sesame) is applied to the back on both sides of the spinal column. Moisturizing cream is unsuitable, as it is absorbed quickly into the skin.

The heel of the hand is pressed into the back as shown, and is rubbed rapidly back and forth, parallel to the spinal column on both sides. Greater pressure should be applied in the upward motion than in the downward one. The friction of the hand on the skin generates heat that is felt by both practitioner and patient. This heat relaxes the muscles and stimulates the circulation and the energy flow in that region.

The rubbing motions should be continued for as long as the patient is able to tolerate the heat and the practitioner is able to maintain the rapid movements without becoming overly tired. If the massage aggravates the existing pain, it should not be continued.

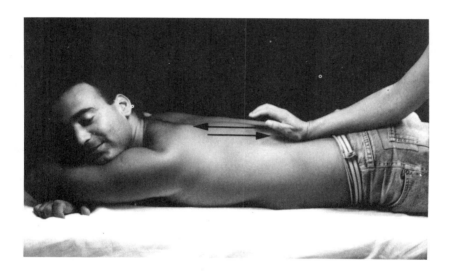

Friction massage

Reflexology

This method of treatment involves using the fingers to massage and press the patient's feet. It is based on the theory which links every internal organ to a specific area of the foot. When a health problem or pain of some sort is present in a given region, we can expect the corresponding site on the foot to be sensitive to pressure.

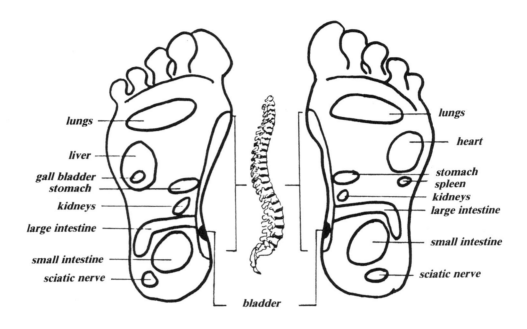

Division of the foot according to internal organs

Reflexology massage has proven itself as a highly effective method of relieving back pain and improving the circulation of the various bodily systems. When utilizing this form of massage to treat the back, it is advisable to go over the entire foot systematically. The treatment involves sliding the thumb over the various regions illustrated below, in the direction of the arrows as shown. Particular time and attention should be devoted to the region of the back. Before beginning the massage, a small amount of oil should be applied to the foot in order to make it easier to slide the thumb over the surface.

Foot massage is an enjoyable form of treatment. It relaxes assorted tensions of which we were previously completely unaware. When the person receiving treatment reports a sensitive spot anywhere along the path of the massage, it is recommended that pressure be applied there. This can be achieved through either a circular or a straight back-and-forth motion over the site. Pressure should not be applied to such a degree that it causes excessive pain.

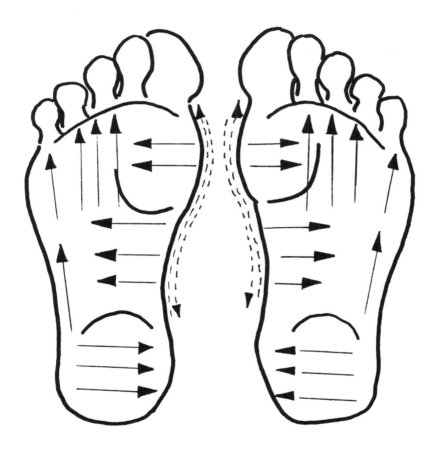

The various directions of foot massage

Compresses

A compress is a source of heat or cold applied to a painful region in order to warm or to cool it. The following are three types of compresses:

A cold compress is recommended immediately after an occurrence of sharp pain resulting from an injury or incorrect movement. A plastic bag containing several ice cubes is applied to the painful site. The cold acts to contract the injured blood vessels in the region, thus reducing the sensation of pain.

A hot compress can consist of a hot water bottle, a towel dipped in hot water or an electric blanket applied to the painful region. This type of compress is recommended in cases of chronic pain. It acts to relax tense muscles, stimulate circulation and improve energy flow in the afflicted area.

A hot compress of medicinal herbs is prepared by boiling 60 grams (4 tablespoons) of fresh ginger root for several minutes in two cups of water. A towel is then dipped in the hot liquid and applied to the painful region. Care should be taken not to apply the towel while the liquid is still too hot, in order to avoid burning the skin. A hot water bottle is placed over the towel.

Another method of relieving pain by heating the afflicted area involves the Chinese medicinal herb, moxa, which can be employed in several ways. The most popular of these is the cigar-shaped "moxa stick" which is lit at one end and used to heat the painful region. The burning end of the stick should be held several centimeters above the skin. It is important to ensure that the person receiving treatment feels a medium level of heat, not too strong and not too weak. The desired length of treatment is 5 to 10 minutes.

Practitioners must be careful to watch the end of the moxa stick continuously until the treatment is completed. Failing to do so can easily lead to a burn on the skin. Every minute or so, the ashes that collect at the end of the stick should be tapped into an ashtray. Proper ventilation of the treatment room is also essential since the burning moxa generates a great deal of smoke. At the conclusion of treatment, the preferred method of extinguishing the flame is by wrapping the head of the "cigar" in aluminum foil in order to cut off the air supply. Putting out the flame by dipping it in water will damage the herb.

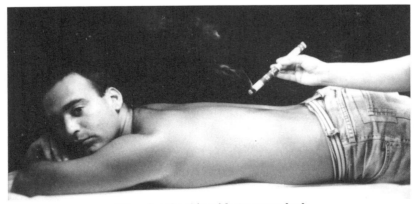

Warming the skin with the moxa herb

Suction Cups

Suction cups are well known as one of "Grandma's remedies," once popular among the older generation. This method of treatment was already practiced in Europe as far back as the Middle Ages. In traditional Chinese medicine, it has been in use for centuries and has retained its popularity today among practitioners of Chinese medicine.

Suction cups act upon the body by creating a vacuum within the cup which has the effect of enhancing circulation and energy flow beneath the skin in the area surrounding the cup. As a result of the vacuum and the destruction of capillaries beneath the treatment site, circles ranging in color from pale red to dark purple appear on the skin where the cups have been applied. (Darker circles simply indicate that a greater amount of blood was previously obstructing circulation and energy flow at the site and has now been dislodged by the treatment.) After a period of one to seven days, these markings will fade completely.

There are a number of ways to create a vacuum inside the cup. The method popular in ancient times involved burning alcohol or paper within the overturned cup. Of course, this practice requires a certain amount of skill and is not recommended for the lay person. Nowadays suction cups come equipped with a manual vacuum pump used for sucking out the air. Anyone can use this type of cup without prior experience.

I would like to dispel here the widespread but misguided notion that suction cups derive their healing power from the heat of the burning fire. The **only** purpose of the fire is to create a vacuum within the cup. The healing effect of the suction cups stems solely from the force of the vacuum created within them.

Periodic treatments with suction cups are recommended for their benefits to the body as a whole. They step up the blood flow and provide a boost to the body's internal energy circulation.

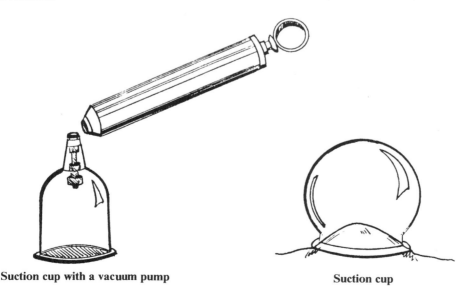

Suction cup with a vacuum pump   **Suction cup**

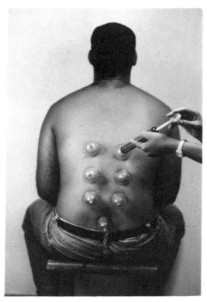

Treatment with suction cups for relief of back pain

Counterindications for the use of suction cups:

- ☐ at the site of a skin disease;
- ☐ at an infected site;
- ☐ at a site with protruding bones (for reasons of pain, and inability to create a vacuum); over the nipples;
- ☐ over the region of the heart;
- ☐ during strong cramps;
- ☐ in the presence of a skin allergy;
- ☐ during an episode of high fever;
- ☐ during pregnancy (due to risk of miscarriage);
- ☐ soon after a previous application of suction cups, while dark markings are still visible on the skin;
- ☐ in patients with a very weak body;
- ☐ in unconscious patients;
- ☐ in infants (due to their extreme sensitivity);
- ☐ with broken or cracked suction cups.

CHAPTER SEVEN

EMOTIONAL FACTORS AND BACK PAIN

"It is our duty to be happy all the time, to overcome and banish the tendency toward sadness and depression in any way possible. All the illnesses that trouble people occur as a result of unhappiness..."

Rabbi Nachman of Bratslav

There is a strong link between chronic pain and emotional states such as depression and tension. Pain can lead to emotional stress and depression while, conversely, tension can manifest itself as physical pain. Pain of the latter type is extremely common nowadays with tension and emotional stress so much a part of the modern lifestyle.

Stress zeroes in on the body's weak points, eventually taking the form of chronic pain. The lower back, because it is subject to constant pressure, represents the ideal site for pain of this type. For this reason, chronic back pain is the most widespread among the range of aches and pains of emotional origin.

Pain that occurs for underlying emotional reasons is actually a cry for help on the part of our subconscious. Other psychological factors then come into play, among them the warmth and attention extended by the "caregiver" towards the "sufferer." Regardless of any emotional factors involved, physical activity is vital in such cases as well, since it has a positive effect on the individual's mental state. The connection between our bodies and our emotions explains why many chronic back-pain sufferers experience a worsening of their condition during periods of stress and depression, even when their pain has been diagnosed as pathological in origin.

CHAPTER EIGHT

EXERCISES FOR THE RELIEF AND PREVENTION OF BACK PAIN

In thousands of cases of back pain, it has been demonstrated that performing the right exercises can bring about significant relief from pain and, in many cases, even eliminate it entirely. Often there is no logical scientific explanation for this, all the more so since back pains occur in the first place for so many different reasons.

The aim of the exercises described below is to alleviate back pain, and to keep the back flexible, strong and in good condition. These exercises do not require fast or strenuous movements, are not tiring and can also be performed by the elderly. Performing these exercises will help in most cases of chronic back pain and sciatica.

Success in overcoming the pain will depend on patient and consistent repetition of the exercises over a lengthy period. The amount of time required to overcome the pain depends on the individual case: the longer your pain has been present, the longer it will take to conquer. Be patient! Overcoming the pain may take several months, but in most cases some improvement will already be noticeable during the first few weeks of exercise. The improvement will occur gradually, and naturally there will be ups and downs over the course of time that you are exercising. For example, progress is slower in the winter than in the summer because the cold causes the muscles to tighten up. Emotional stress can also slow down your progress. The usual pattern of improvement that can be expected is expressed in the following graph, which indicates rises and falls in the rate of progress as part of an overall upward trend towards improvement.

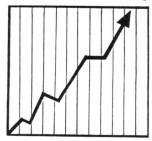

Many people who are accustomed to engaging in sports invest a lot of effort in keeping up with their regular routine despite the fact that they are experiencing back pain. It is essential in such cases to take a break from your regular sports activities in order to avoid stretching of the muscles and unnecessary pressure on them, two factors which are liable to aggravate the pain and to greatly retard the healing process. Swimming is recommended as an intermediate solution, since it does not cause unnecessary pressure on the vertebrae and can even help greatly in relieving back pain. However, there are cases where swimming actually aggravates an existing condition. In such situations, swimming must be discontinued for a period of time, even if it has been one of your regular activities until now.

Remember that the goal of these exercises is to overcome back pain. You don't have to demonstrate acrobatic ability. You are not in competition with others — not even with yourself. You are coping here with pain! The struggle must be a persistent and non-aggressive one. **Avoid performing exercises that cause you pain!** The back is an extremely fragile and sensitive region, and must be treated with delicacy and understanding. Learn to know your back — what causes it pain and what brings it comfort. Don't strain it unnecessarily. Treat it gently and with tolerance.

Perform only those exercises which do not cause you pain. If you can only perform a particular exercise painlessly in one direction, be sure to limit yourself to that direction alone, even if this gives you a feeling of "asymmetry." The best time to perform the exercises is in the morning, right after awakening and while still on an empty stomach. Make sure to match your breathing to the exercises according to the instructions given. **Your respiratory functions are an inseparable part of your physical activity, and an important factor linking the interior and the exterior of the body.** After every few exercises, be sure to assume one of the Relaxation Positions for several minutes (see following section).

Make it a point to do the exercises every day! Many people, after exercising for a certain length of time, begin to feel some relief from their pain and tend to become lazy about performing the exercises on a regular, daily basis. This is a dangerous course of action, and one that is liable to worsen your condition. Remind yourself how important it is to stick with it! You need to be patient and give your body time to change from within, to become stronger and more flexible. Avoid getting drawn into feelings of self-pity, frustration and depression. View this program of daily exercise as a start towards solving your problem, and with persistence your success is guaranteed!

The exercises that appear on the following pages are of varying levels of difficulty. Try to select for yourself those exercises that you find most comfortable. Begin slowly, and don't try to jump right into performing "impressive" movements. After several weeks or months, when your ability has improved, you can choose from a broader range of exercises.

Taking care of your body is something that cannot be put off. Make this effort a part of your daily routine or you will never find the time to do it. So from this moment on, look after your body and its flexibility on a daily basis. Pay attention to your body, exercise its muscles, activate its energy channels and save yourself pain and suffering. The following exercises will give you an additional daily bonus of enjoyment, vitality and life enhancement, and will help keep your body in good condition. They will improve the quality of your life, and slow down the aging process.

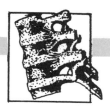

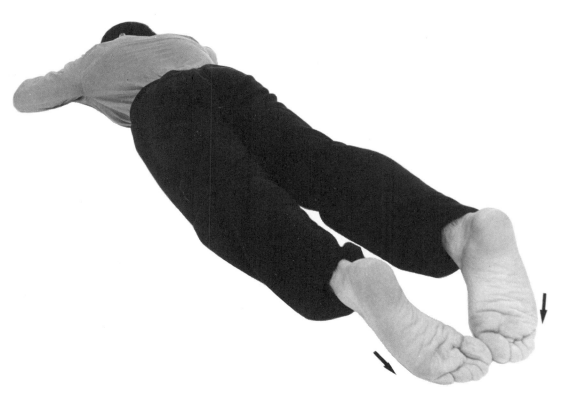

RELAXATION POSITION 1

Lie on your stomach. Raise your pelvic region by placing a pillow under it.

1 Lay your head on your hands.
2 Point your big toes inward so that they touch each other.
3 Remain in this position for several minutes.

"He who often hurries will often fail."

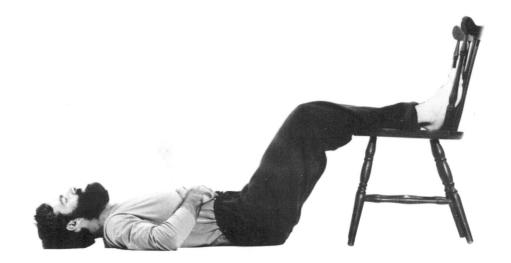

RELAXATION POSITION 2

Lie on your back.

1 Rest your legs on a chair as shown in the photo.

2 Remain in this position for several minutes.

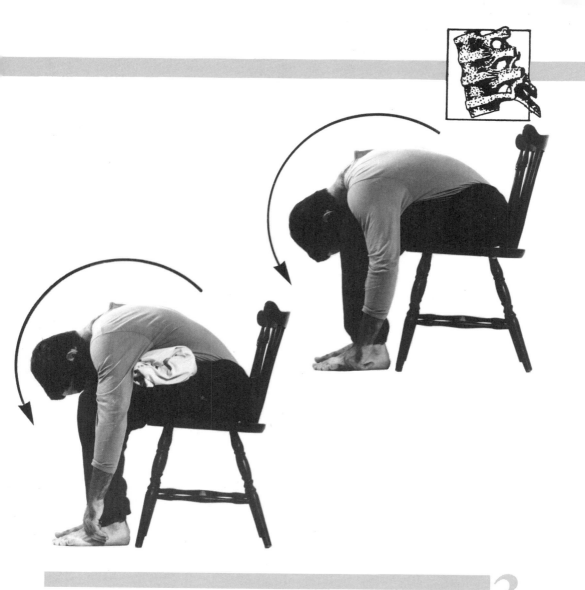

RELAXATION POSITION 3

Sit on a chair.

1 Bend foward, and rest your shoulders and chest on your knees.

2 Relax the muscles of your body as much as possible, and remain in this position for one or two minutes.

If you are unable to rest your chest on your knees comfortably, support yourself with a large pillow between your chest and knees as shown in the photo.

"Moderacy is the guiding light of science."

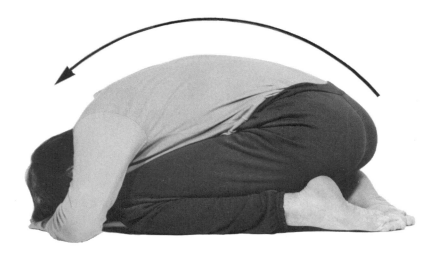

RELAXATION POSITION 4

Kneel down.

1 Bend forward and relax the muscles of your body as much as possible.

It is important to assume this position after performing any exercises that involve bending backwards.

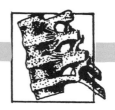

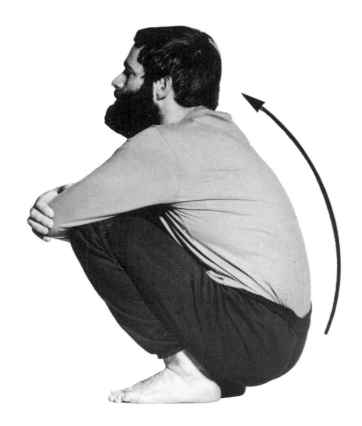

RELAXATION POSITION 5

Sit as shown in the photo.

1 Make sure to place the heels firmly on the floor.

2 Remain in this position for several minutes.

"To ask, is a moment's shame.
Not to ask, is the shame of a lifetime."

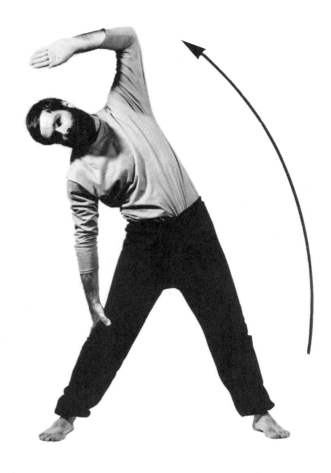

BACK EXERCISE 1

Stand straight, with your legs spread apart.

1 Raise your right arm, bending the elbow above your head. While exhaling, bend your body to the left until your left hand touches your thigh.

2 Remain in this position without breathing for 3 to 5 seconds.

3 Return to the original upright position while inhaling.

4 Repeat this exercise three times on each side, alternating the direction.

If bending the back in a given direction causes pain, do this exercise only toward the other side. Make sure to extend the elbow backwards.

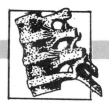

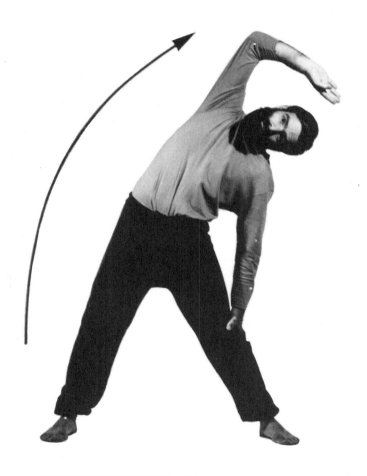

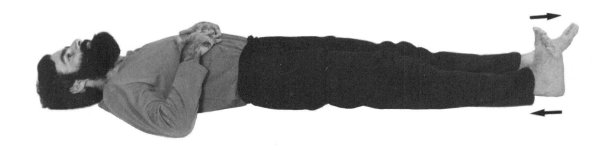

BACK EXERCISE 2

Lie on your back.

1 While exhaling, stretch your feet in opposite directions (one flexed, the other extended).

2 Maintain this position for 3 to 5 seconds.

3 Relax the feet, and repeat the above with a change in direction.

4 Repeat this exercise 6 to 10 times.

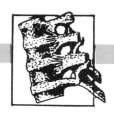

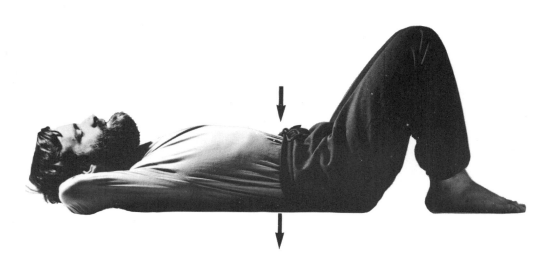

BACK EXERCISE 3

Lie on your back with your knees bent.

1 While exhaling, press your lower back firmly to the floor.
2 Remain in this position without breathing for 3 to 5 seconds.
3 Relax the pressure as you inhale.
4 Repeat this exercise 3 to 6 times.

"Consistency is of prime importance."

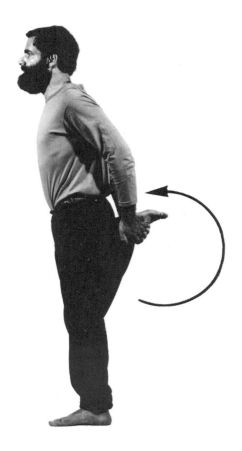

BACK EXERCISE 4

Stand up straight.

1 Place your knees so that your thighs line up as closely as possible. While exhaling, draw your left heel up to your buttocks.

2 Remain in this position for 3 to 5 seconds.

3 Release your ankle while inhaling, and return to the original position.

4 Repeat this exercise 3 times on each side.

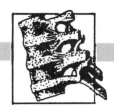

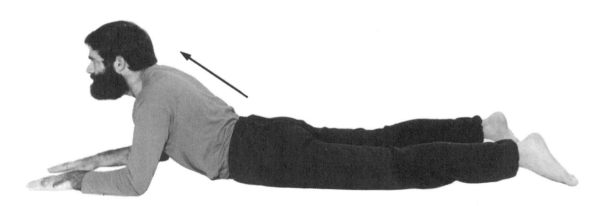

BACK EXERCISE 5

Lie on your stomach.

1 Lean on your elbows, and concentrate on relaxing the muscles of your back as much as possible.

2 Remain in this position for 30 to 60 seconds.

"He who hurries will fail due to his haste, while he who is careful will succeed due to his caution."

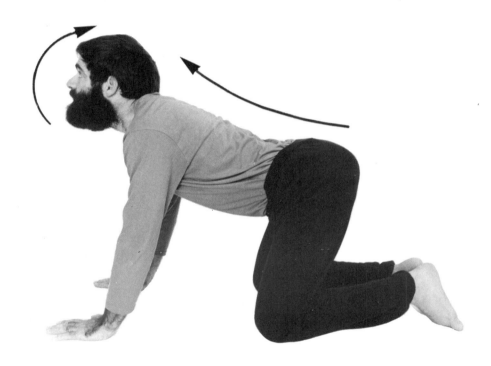

BACK EXERCISE 6

Kneel on all fours.

1 Raise your head and push your stomach outwards and down towards the floor as you inhale. Make sure to focus your eyes on the highest point in the room.

2 Bend your head inwards, towards your chest, as you round your back upwards and exhale.

3 Repeat the exercise 10-15 times.

If the upward or downward motion of your head causes pain in the neck area, then move your head only slightly — until just before the point where the pain occurs. Perform the exercise as slowly as possible.

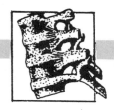

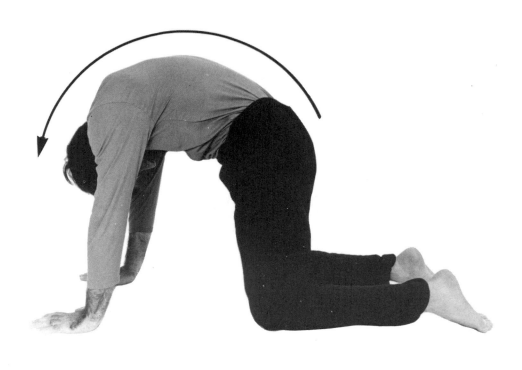

"*Every generation laughs at the old-fashioned while becoming slaves to the new.*"

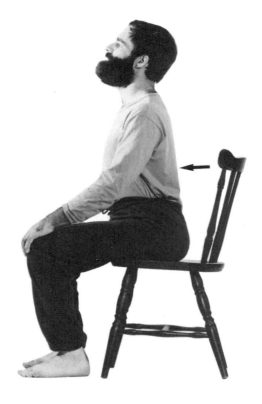

BACK EXERCISE 7

Sit on a chair without leaning back. Rest your hands on your knees.

1 Stretch your shoulders back and chest out while inhaling. Remain in this position for 1 to 2 seconds.

2 Relax your chest and shoulders while exhaling.

3 Repeat this exercise 5 to 10 times.

Make sure to perform the exercise slowly. This exercise is excellent for people who spend many hours daily in a sitting position. It should be performed every so often during the day.

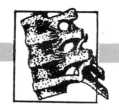

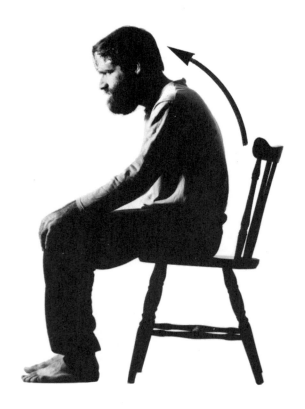

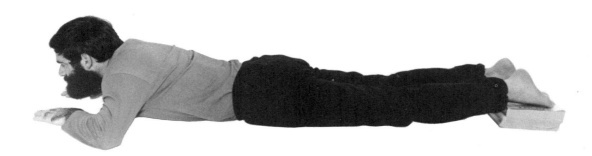

BACK EXERCISE 8

Lie on your stomach, resting your feet on several books at a height of 10 to 15 cm. off the floor.

1 Raise the pelvic region while exhaling.
2 Hold this position for 3 to 5 seconds, then relax.
3 Repeat this exercise 3 to 6 times.

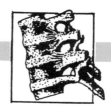

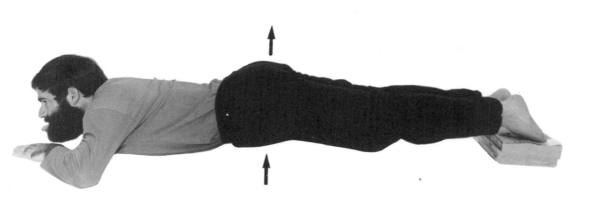

"*Idleness is more tiring than exertion.*"

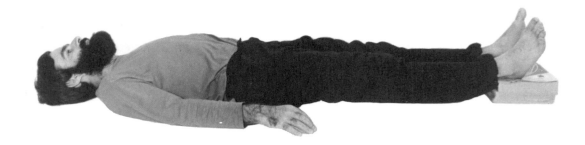

BACK EXERCISE 9

Lie on your back. Rest your heels on several books at a height of 10 to 15 cm. off the floor.

1 Raise the pelvic region while exhaling.
2 Hold this position for 3 to 5 seconds, then relax.
3 Repeat this exercise 3 to 6 times.

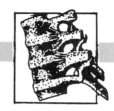

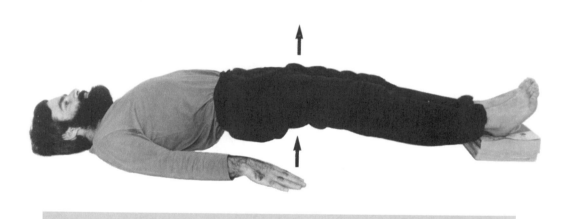

"*Relief from pain is achieved through persistence,
gentleness, understanding and patience.*"

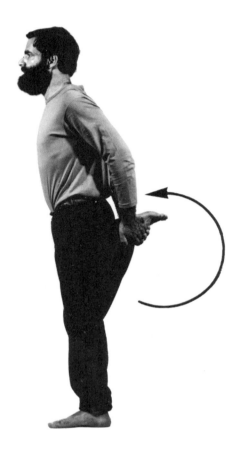

BACK EXERCISE 10

Stand on one leg (as in Exercise 4).

1 Extend the bent leg backward while exhaling, and lean your upper torso forward.

2 Remain in this position for 3 to 10 seconds.

3 Relax and return to the upright position.

4 Repeat the exercise 3 times on each side, alternating each time.

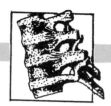

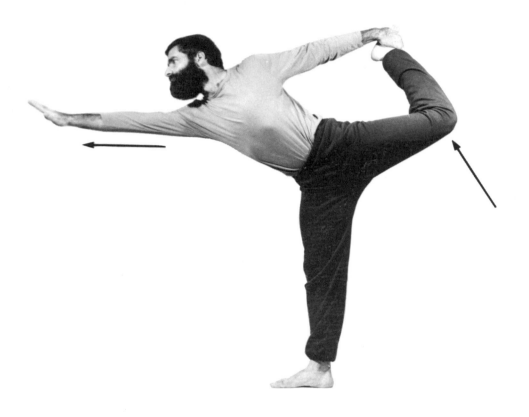

When performing this exercise, use a chair or wall for support. Be careful not to overstretch your muscles. If you feel tension behind the knee of the straight leg — even if your extended thigh is not completely parallel to the floor — you should stop for now. With time and persistence, your ability to perform this exercise will improve.

"Nature grants us nothing without hard work."

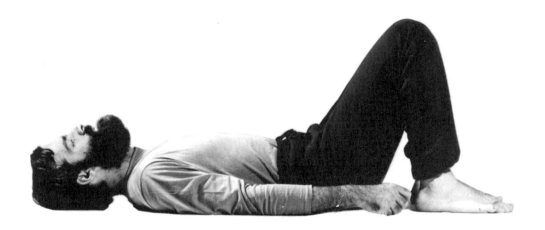

BACK EXERCISE 11

Lie on your back with knees bent.

1. While exhaling, raise your buttocks as shown in the photo and hold this position for 5 to 10 seconds.
2. Repeat this exercise 3 to 6 times.

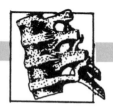

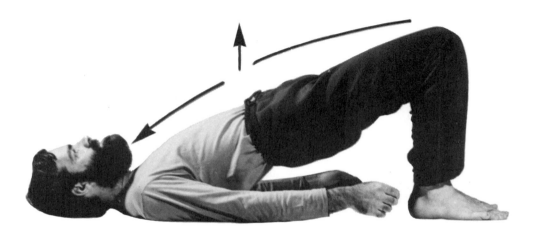

*"If your goal cannot be achieved through
moderation, how can it be achieved at all?"*

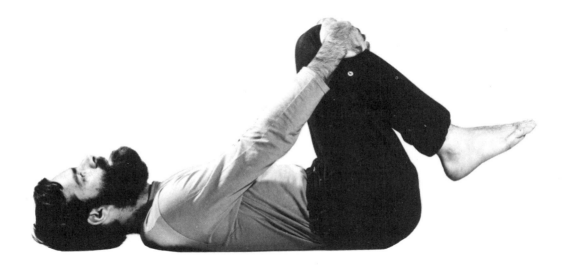

BACK EXERCISE 12

Lie on your back, grasping your knees with your hands.

1. Draw your knees up toward your chest while exhaling.
2. Remain in this position for 5 seconds.
3. Relax, returning to your original position.
4. Repeat this exercise 3 to 6 times.

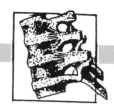

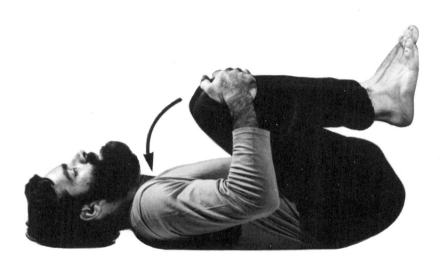

"He who is lazy only increases his weakness."

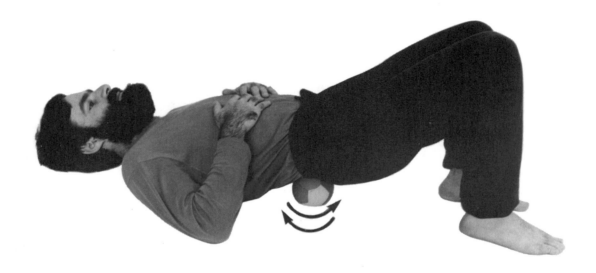

BACK EXERCISE 13

Lie on your back. Raise your buttocks and place a tennis or other soft ball underneath your waist.

1 Without bringing your full weight to bear on the ball, perform circular motions with the lower portion of your body, using the ball as a central axis.

2 Perform 10 to 20 circular motions, both clockwise and counterclockwise.

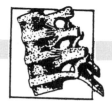

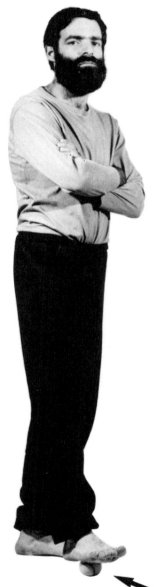

BACK EXERCISE 14

Stand or sit, as you prefer.

1 Place a tennis ball on the floor, underneath your foot as shown.

2 Massage your foot by applying pressure to the ball for 2 to 3 minutes. Perform the massage on your other foot as well.

This massage stimulates circulation in the foot and relaxes the leg muscles. It also helps relax the muscles of the back.

"Stay far away from doubt."

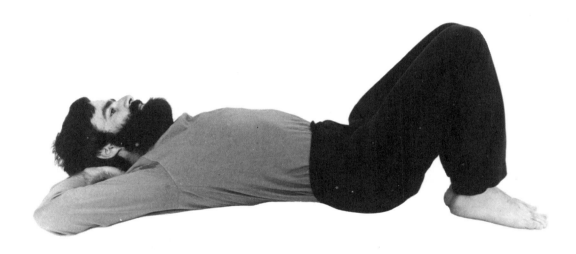

BACK EXERCISE 15

Lie on your back. Bend your knees, keeping them together. Fold your arms under the back of your neck.

1 As you exhale, lean your knees to the right while keeping them together, and touch them to the floor.

2 Remain in this position for 1 to 2 seconds. Return to your original position while inhaling.

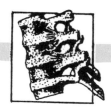

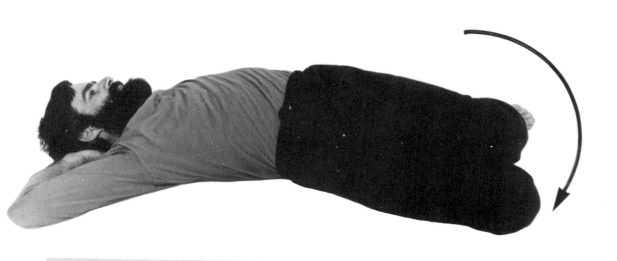

3 Perform this exercise 3 times in each
direction, alternating sides.

If you feel pain when performing this
exercise in a given direction, do it only on
the other side.

"Prevention is the root of all healing."

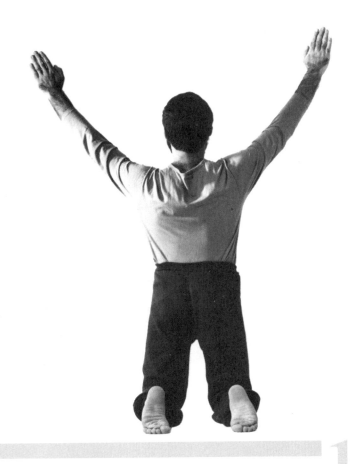

BACK EXERCISE 16

Kneel down, raising your arms.

1 While exhaling, turn slowly to your right, and touch your left heel with your right hand.

2 Maintain this position for 1 to 2 seconds.

3 Return to your original position while inhaling.

4 Repeat this exercise 10 to 15 times in each direction, alternating sides.

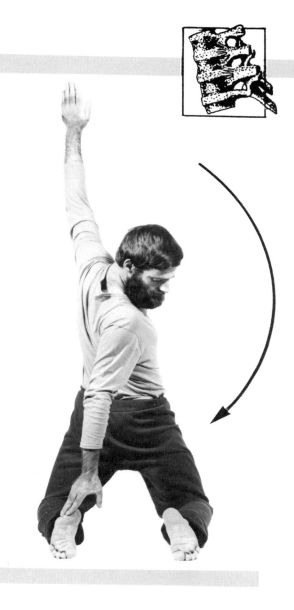

Make certain to look at your heels as you touch them. If performing this exercise in a given direction causes pain, do it only toward the other side.

"If we follow nature's path, we cannot stray."

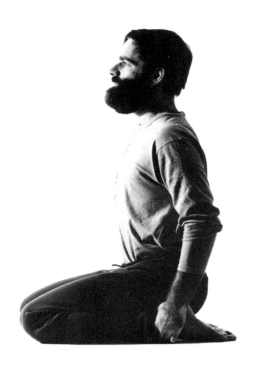

BACK EXERCISE

Kneel as shown in the photo and grasp your ankles.

1 Raise yourself up slowly, and stretch your shoulders backwards while inhaling.

2 Maintain this position for 1 to 2 seconds, then relax and return to your original position.

3 Repeat this exercise 5 to 10 times.

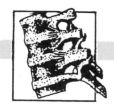

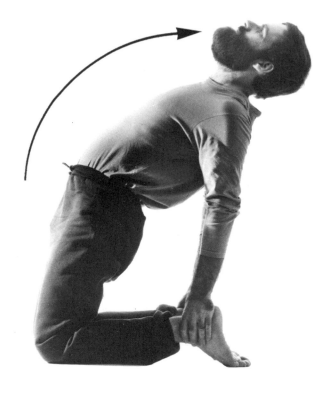

"Habits are second nature."

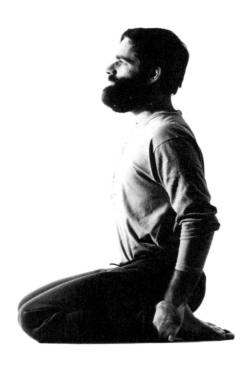

BACK EXERCISE 18

Kneel as shown in the photo and grasp your ankles.

1 While exhaling, bend backwards until you are leaning on your elbows.

2 While breathing lightly, hold this position for 10 to 20 seconds, or as long as you feel comfortable.

3 Return to your original position, and immediately switch to Relaxation Position 4 (see page 42).

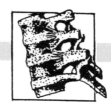

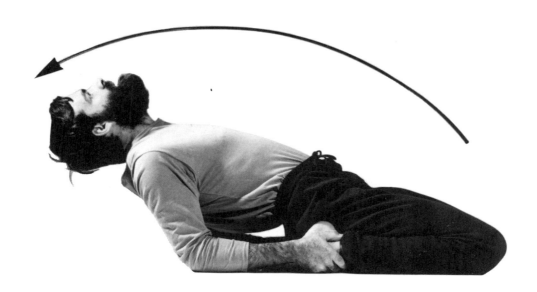

"He who wishes to succeed in important matters must
pay careful attention to unimportant ones."

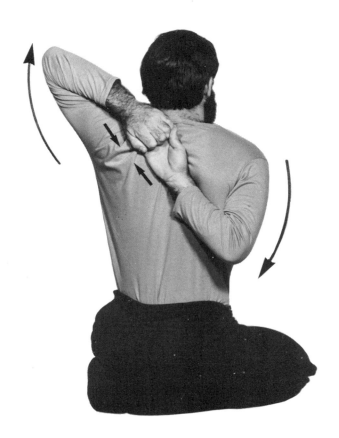

BACK EXERCISE 19

Sit or stand, as you prefer.

1 Raise one hand over your shoulder and the other behind your back.

2 Stretch your elbow backwards, and straighten your back as much as possible.

3 Remain in this position for 10 to 30 seconds while breathing slowly and quietly.

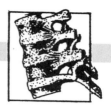

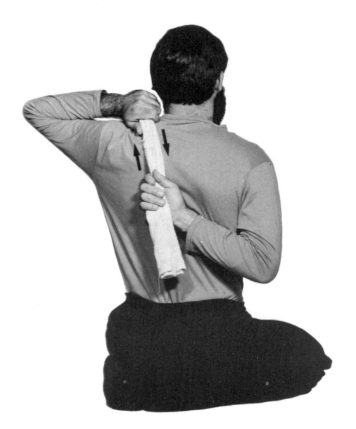

4 Perform this exercise three times on each side, alternating the direction.

For the first few weeks, it is advisable to use a towel when performing this exercise until you have achieved sufficient flexibility for your hands to grasp one another. Make sure that you don't overstretch your muscles.

"Be forceful yet gentle."

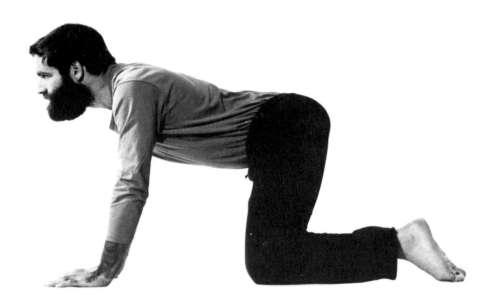

BACK EXERCISE 20

Lean on your hands and knees.

1 While exhaling, lift your left leg until it is parallel to the floor, keeping your leg straight.

2 Remain in this position for 5 to 10 seconds, then relax.

3 Perform this exercise 3 times on each side, alternating the direction.

If you feel pain on a given side when performing this exercise, do it only on the other side.

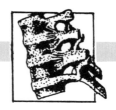

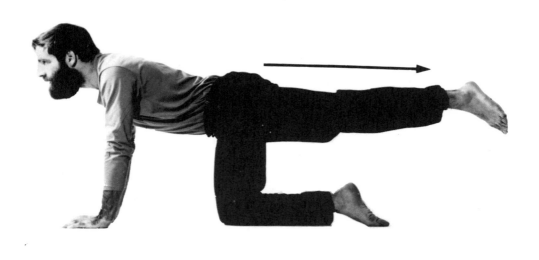

"Wealth is the absence of pain.'

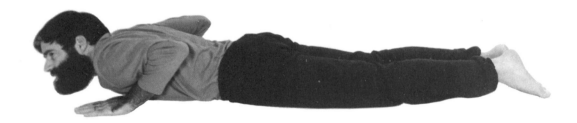

BACK EXERCISE 21

Lie on your stomach.

1 While inhaling, raise your chest slowly by pressing your hands against the floor, and look up at the ceiling.

2 Remain in this position for 3 to 5 seconds, returning slowly to your original position as you exhale.

3 Perform this exercise 3 to 6 times.

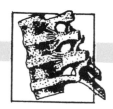

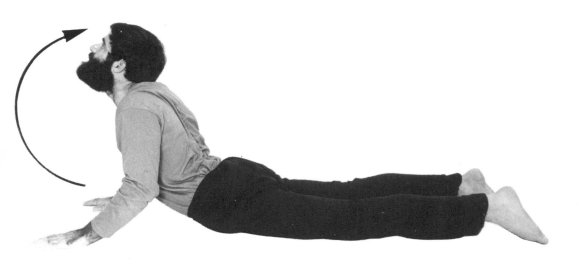

When performing this exercise, be careful not to raise your hips off the floor. Make sure to keep your elbows as close to your body as possible.

"Only action will bring vitality to your life."

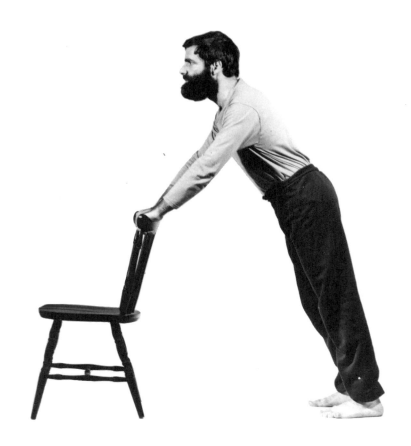

BACK EXERCISE 22

Lean on a chair.

1 While exhaling, lean your body forward, making sure that your heels remain in contact with the floor.

2 When you begin to feel a slight tension behind your knees, hold your position for 5 to 10 seconds while breathing lightly.

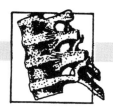

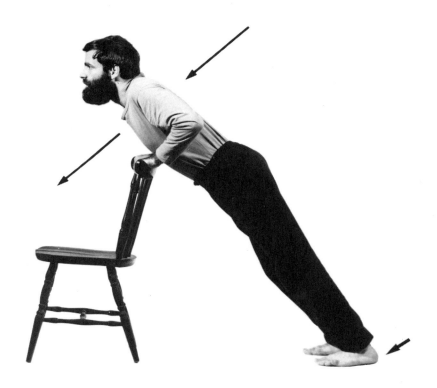

3 Relax and return to your original
position as you inhale. Repeat this
exercise 5 to 10 times.

"Don't wait for others to do your work for you."

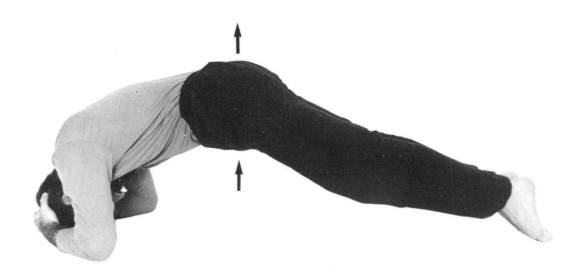

BACK EXERCISE 23

Link the fingers of both hands together behind your head. Rest the crown of your head on the floor, with hips and thighs raised as shown in the photo.
Important! The weight of the upper part of your body should rest on your elbows, not your head.

1 While exhaling, lower your hips very slowly toward the floor until you feel a slight tension in the muscles at the nape of your neck.

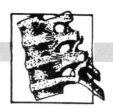

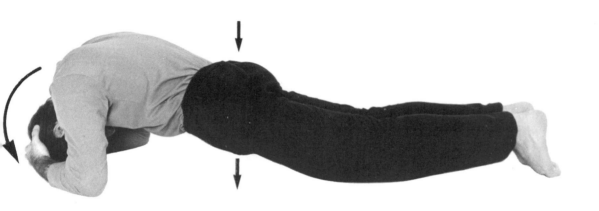

2 Hold this position for 2 to 3 seconds.

3 Return to your original position while inhaling. Repeat this exercise 3 times.

4 Gradually increase the number of bends to between 6 and 10.

After performing this exercise, shift immediately to Relaxation Position 1. During this exercise, the hips should not be lowered beyond the point where you feel a slight sense of tension at the back of your neck. People who suffer from neck problems must refrain from performing this exercise. If the exercise causes any pain whatsoever, it should not be performed.

"He who rides swiftly is not safe from obstacles along the way."

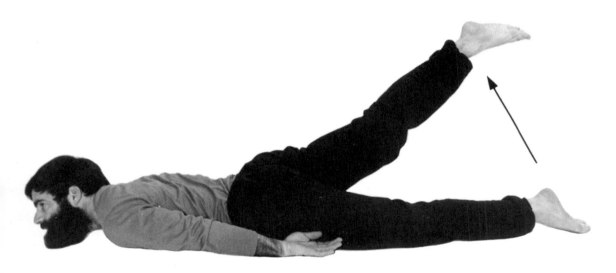

BACK EXERCISE 24

Lie on your stomach, with your hands placed palms up alongside your body.

1 As you exhale, raise your right leg as high as is comfortably possible, keeping the leg straight.

2 Remain in this position for 3 to 5 seconds.

3 Lower the leg while inhaling.

4 Repeat this exercise three times on each side, alternating sides.

If performing this exercise causes you pain on a given side, do it only on the side that doesn't hurt.

CHAPTER NINE

ACQUIRING HEALTHY HABITS

"Man is by nature a creature of habit."
Maimonides

Correct posture prevents tension in the muscles and unnecessary pressure on the spinal column, and is just as important as the system of exercises offered on the preceding pages for relieving back pain.

The cardinal rule in maintaining correct posture is to **keep your back straight**. Good back posture is linked with the lordosis, the medical term for the normal curvature, or indentation, of the lower spine. As long as we keep this indentation in its natural position, we remain comfortable by avoiding excessive pressure on the lower vertebrae. In many cases, this practice is sufficient to prevent the occurrence of pain. If this balance is disturbed and the lordosis becomes rounded, a state of pressure is created, which in turn leads to pain.

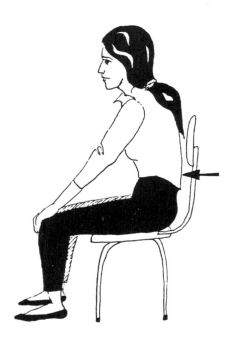

Lordosis rounded-pain

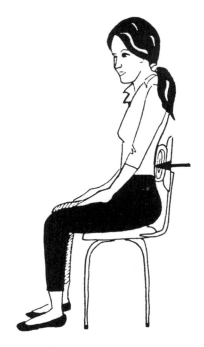

Lordosis intact — no pain

It is particularly important to maintain the correct shape of the lordosis when sitting, as this position exerts intense pressure on the lower portion of the spinal column. By getting into the habit of preserving the lordosis when sitting down or rising from a chair, we can significantly reduce the incidence of many types of back pain. Adhering to this simple rule of keeping your back straight can generate almost instant results, even in acute episodes of severe back pain. It is not easy to adopt new habits of posture and movement. You must learn to pay attention to the position of your body and to constantly remind yourself to improve your posture. The stricter you are about following these rules, the better you'll feel. And eventually, your new habits will become second nature.

Chairs: Sitting Down, Getting Up

1. Stand up straight, as close as possible to the chair.
2. Bend your knees, and sit on the forward part of the chair without leaning back.

Be careful not to lean your body weight forward as you bend your knees! In order to accomplish this, use only your thigh muscles. After you've sat down, remember to keep your back straight and to maintain correct lordosis position.

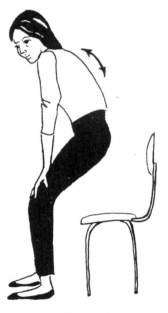

Incorrect

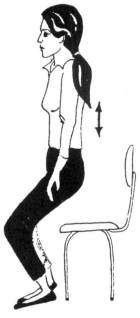

Correct

To return to a standing position, reverse the above procedure, and stand on your feet using your thigh muscles without bending your body weight forward.

Try to sit on chairs with a strong, firm back. Avoid sitting in armchairs or other heavily upholstered seats. Soft upholstery makes it difficult to maintain the lordosis, impairs balance in posture, and increases your chances of pain.

Sitting in a Car

When we drive, there is a tendency to hunch forward and curve our back. This is an unhealthy position that harms balance and posture, eliminates the lordosis and makes us more susceptible to pain. In order to avoid back pain caused by sitting in a car, try to sit straight on the seat. Nowadays, car accessory stores carry special backrests that help to maintain an upright seating position. Another option is to fill the space between the seatback and your lower back with a folded towel or small cushion, as we illustrated earlier with regard to sitting on a regular chair. On the seat itself, you can place a cushion, a thick book or any other firm surface that will prevent your posterior from sinking into the seat.

Working in an Office

Many people spend the bulk of their waking hours working at a desk, facing a computer screen, talking on the telephone or sitting in lengthy meetings. It is important to apply correct habits throughout your workday. Make sure that you have a suitable chair and sit close to your desk or table. The desk should be of proper height in relation to the chair so as to enable you to keep your back upright. If your chair is too high for you, it is advisable to use a footrest in order to rest your feet more firmly and keep your thighs at a suitable height.

Lying Down

Try to sleep on a firm mattress. There are types of mattresses available on the market today that are recommended for their "special adaptability to the body." Not all of these are suitable for individuals who suffer from back pain. If you feel discomfort when lying on your mattress, experiment for a time with sleeping on several blankets spread on the floor.

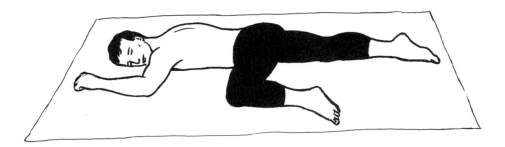

The most natural sleeping position is on your side with one knee raised. If you find it uncomfortable to lie on your side and are used to falling asleep on your back, fill the space underneath your neck with a rolled-up towel and place large pillows under your legs, as shown. For your neck, it is advisable to use a special cushion known as a cervical pillow. These can be obtained at pharmacies and stores that carry medical accessories.

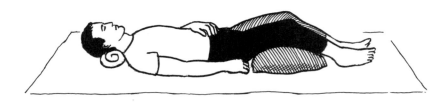

If you are accustomed to falling asleep only on your stomach, but this position is painful, try placing a pillow under your pelvic region. This will raise your posterior and reduce unnecessary pressure on the lower vertebrae.

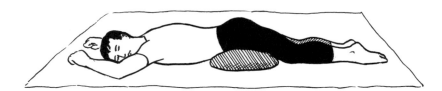

Movement

Avoid performing any motions that cause pain, as these are likely to worsen your condition and hamper improvement. Stay away from sports involving rapid, sharp or strenuous movements. Activities such as running, jumping rope, weightlifting, cycling, and riding an "exercycle" are not recommended for individuals who suffer from back pain.

Lifting Objects

Avoid lifting heavy objects. Even when lifting light things off the floor, be careful not to bend your back to reach the object. When lifting something from the floor, it is important to keep your back straight and knees bent. The correct way to lift objects is by using the leg rather than the back muscles.

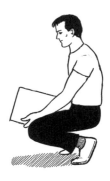

Correct

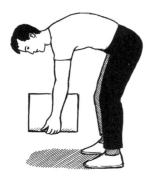

Incorrect

Shoes and Arch Supports

High-heeled shoes should be avoided. The raised heel impairs the body's balance, thus generating tension in the back muscles. The position of the foot is vital to correct posture. Flat feet can sometimes be the reason behind back pain. In such a case, arch supports offer an efficient solution. If you have a tendency toward flat feet, it is advisable to see an orthopedist who can fit you with custom-made arch supports.

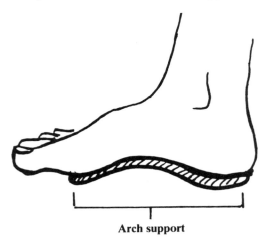

Arch support

Air Conditioning

Cold generally has a negative effect on chronic back pain since its "penetrating" quality causes contraction of the muscles. In addition, cold air blocks the flow of energy through its designated channels (known as meridians), thus encouraging the development of various rheumatic and joint pains. For these reasons, individuals who suffer from back pain, or who have a tendency toward pains in the joints, should avoid air-conditioned settings whenever possible.

A FEW WORDS ON CORRECT NUTRITION

"Strength is gained not from the food you give your body,
but from what your body absorbs of this nourishment."

Aristotle

People invest a great deal of money and effort in their cars because they know that the wrong type of oil or gas for their model can cause damage to the motor; yet these same people are so quick to neglect the most important machines of all — their bodies. Modern man treats his body as if it were a garbage can to be filled with bad food and poisonous cigarette smoke. Fortunately our bodies, unlike cars, are equipped with a dynamic system capable of repairing and renewing itself. This ability diminishes with advancing age. For this reason, a young person can survive on poor-quality food without feeling any immediate damage. In contrast, older people are forced to maintain careful eating habits since their stomachs are weak and cannot digest certain foods.

Food builds our bodies. The digestive process breaks down our food, extracting from it basic substances and energy that serve to build up the body and maintain it. A body that is fed bad food nets a poor return on the energy it has to invest in breaking down that food. The result is a state of overall weakness that ultimately puts the body at risk for various illnesses and pains.

Numerous illnesses and disorders stem from poor eating habits. In a great many cases, a successful cure depends on correcting bad nutritional habits and instituting a proper diet. It is advisable to make things easier for your body by eating good-quality, easily digestible foods that will supply energy and minerals in the necessary amounts.

The underlying reason for many rheumatic and arthritic problems is weakness of the body's excretory systems. Uric acid deposits and other poisonous substances accumulate in the muscles and joints, leading to pain attacks. Thus the recovery process must include bolstering the excretory systems through nutritional means in order to rid ourselves of waste deposits as rapidly as possible.

To find an acupuncturist or doctor of Chinese medicine in your area, contact the following organizations:

American Association of Acupuncture and Oriental Medicine
4101 Lake Bone Trail #201
Raleigh, NC 27607
(919) 787-5181

National Commission for the Certification of Acupuncturists
c/o National Acupuncture Headquarters
1424 16th St. NW, Suite 501
Washington, DC 20036
(202) 232-1404